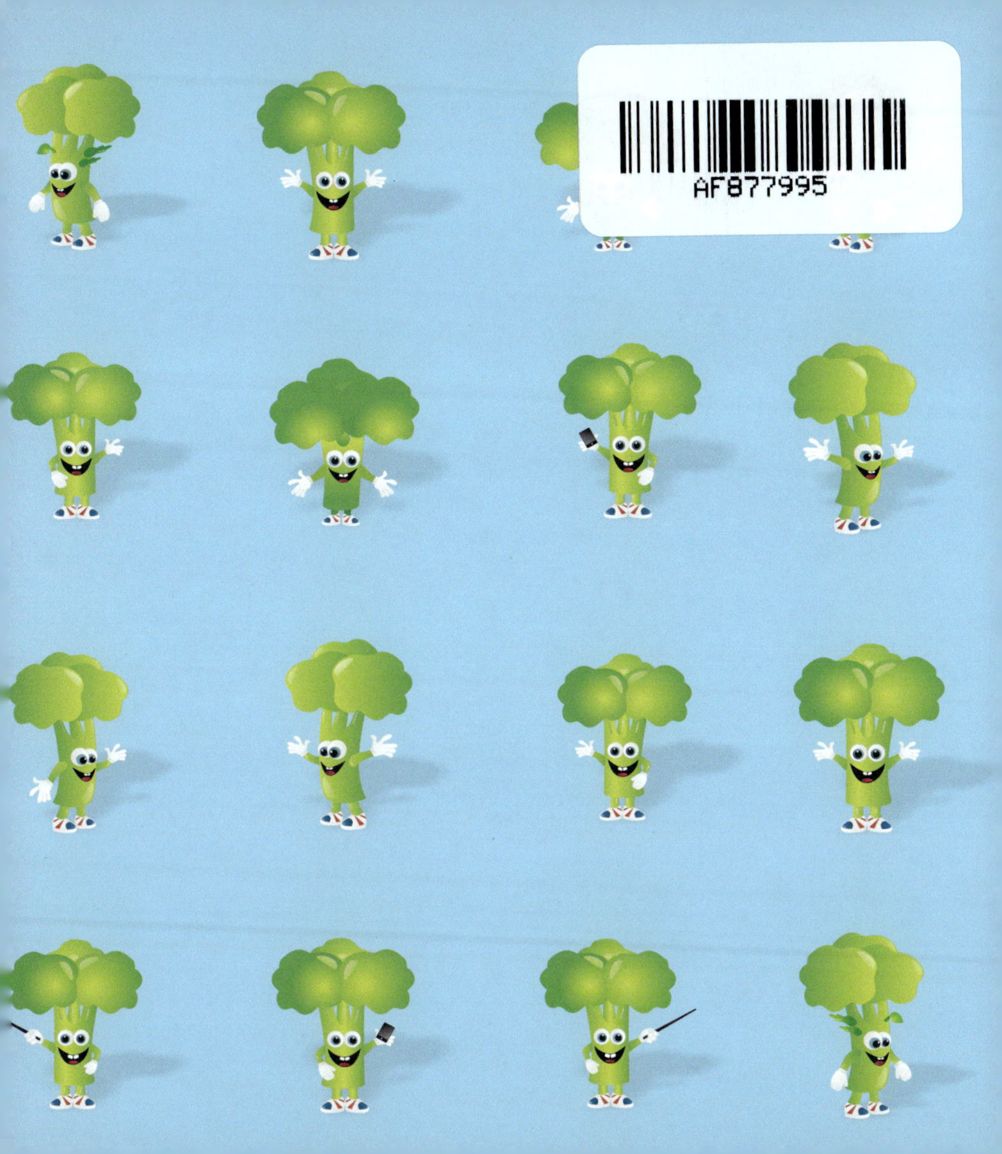

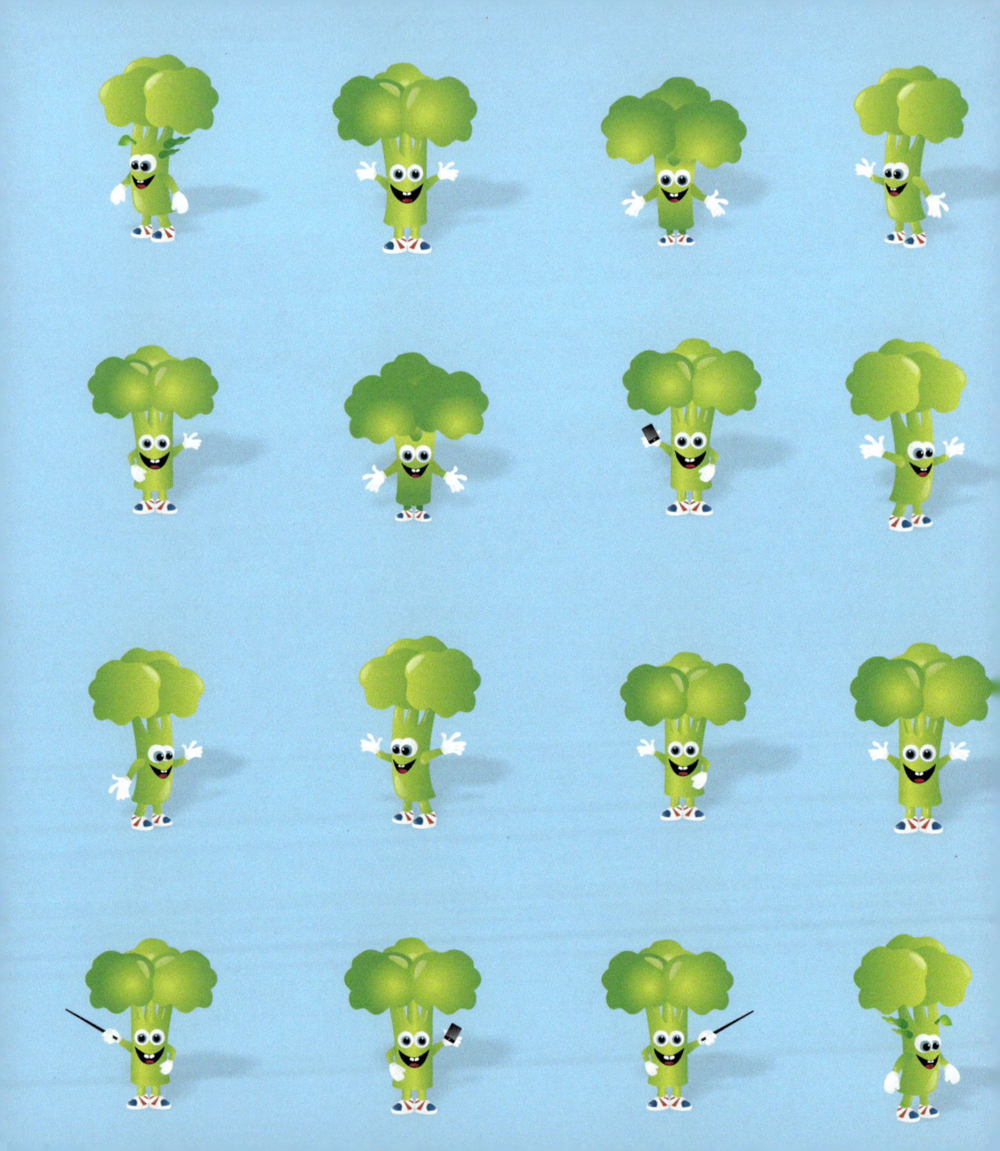

MEET PAULY

by Ana Divo

Illustrated
by Jose Divo

Centecorp Publishing
Orlando, Florida, USA

"To my son Isaac, with all my love"

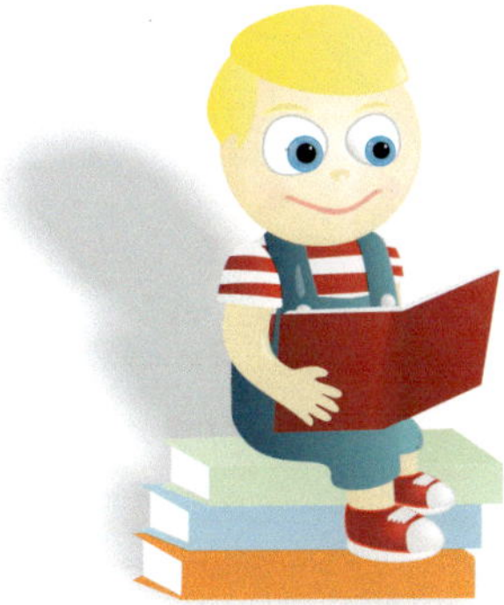

A Note from the Author:

As a mom with a desire to feed my child with organic healthy foods, I tried to make eating a fun learning experience by creating little edible friends.

Reading the story of each character while having a good time teaching our children true facts about each one of these little food friends makes for a fun and healthy start.

A balanced diet is important for the child's body, brain, and functional development. Make a difference from an early age in your children's eating habits by helping them get all the nutrients, vitamins, and minerals they need to enjoy a healthy life.

Have your children Love and Learn about good food. Encourage them to grow strong and healthy with the help of all our little friends from The Organic Learning Adventure Collection.

Bon Appétit!

I have a broccoli friend, his name is Pauly.
He makes me laugh. Oh, he's so jolly!
He's cute, small and a little chubby.
He is delightful in my tummy!

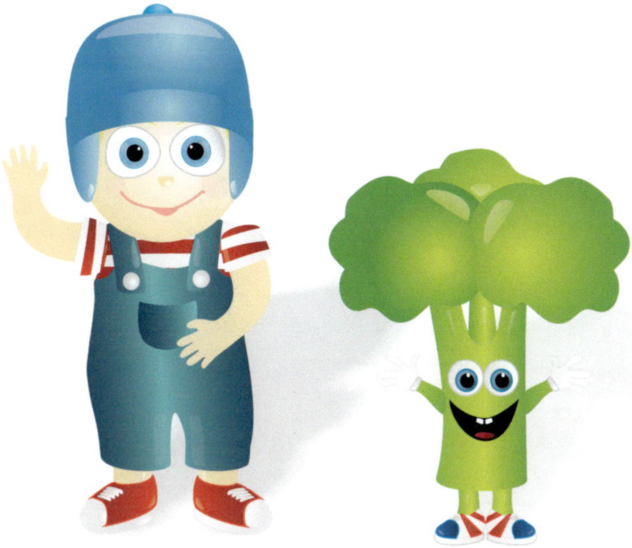

This tasty little guy has a big flower head.
"He looks so funny"
my daddy said...

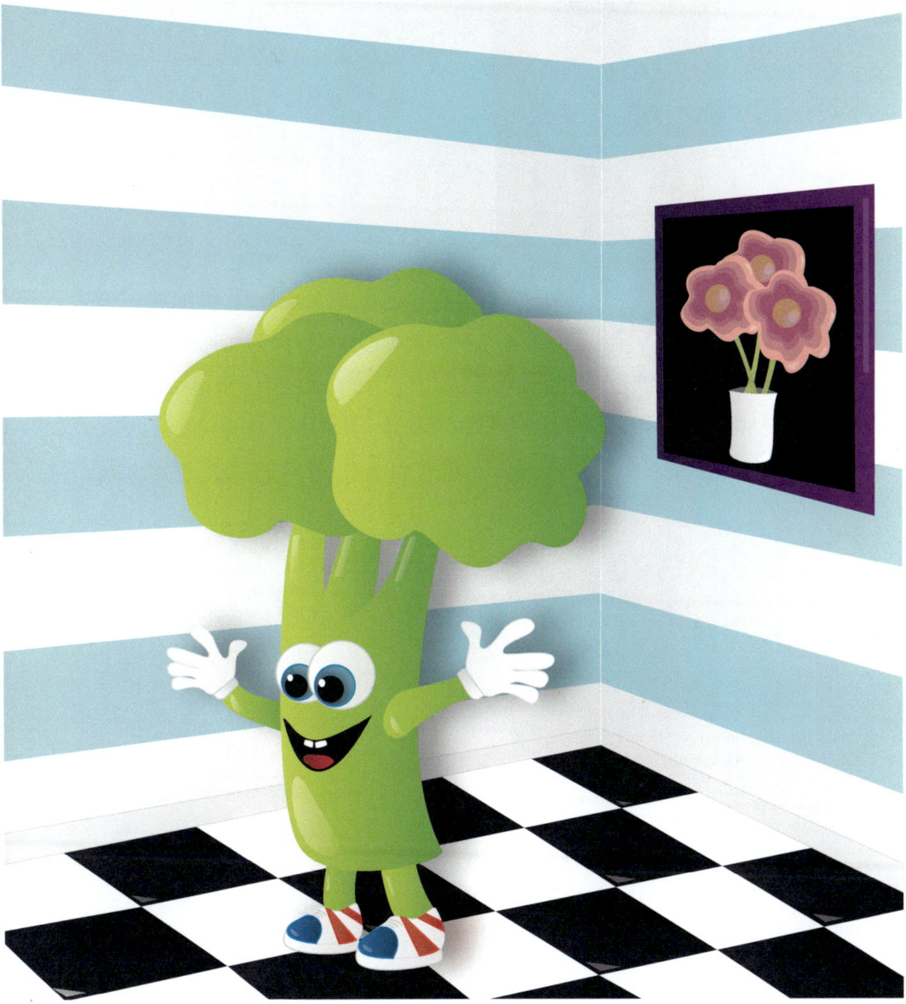

My Broccoli friend is green,
he reminds me of a tree I've seen.
He has branches sprouting from a stalk,
and leaves that move when he goes for a walk.

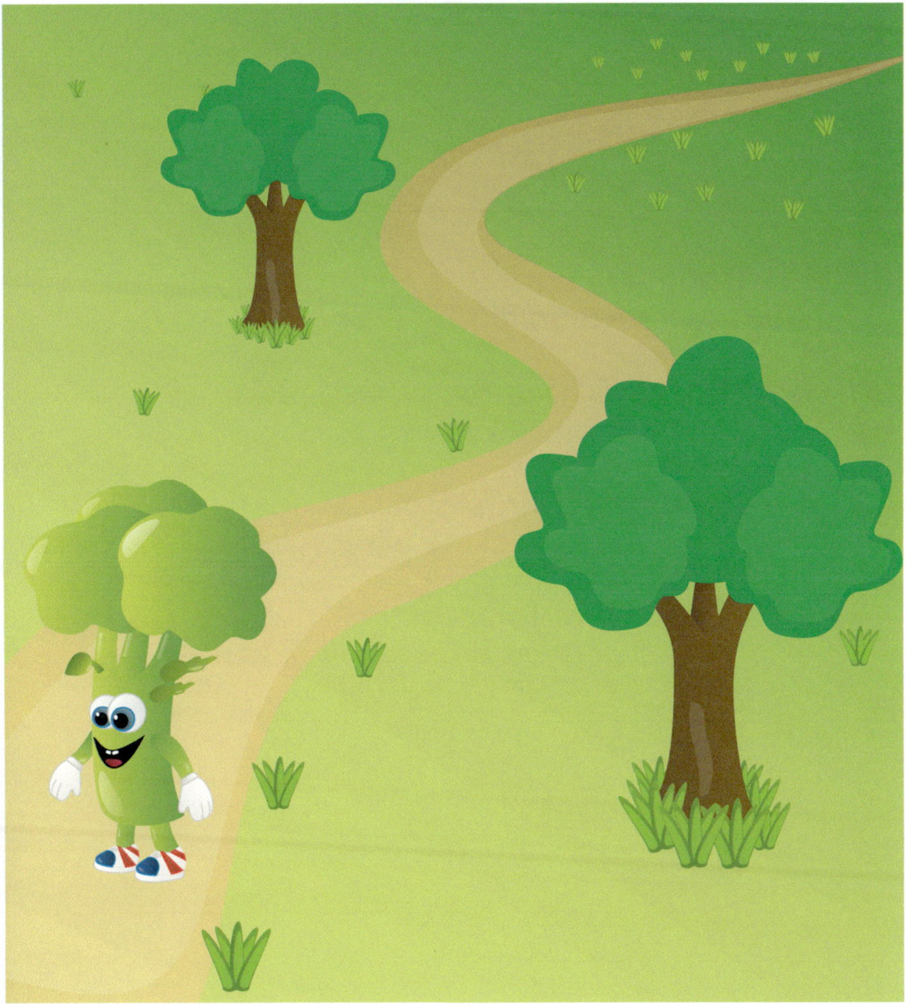

Pauly was born in a California valley
surrounded by rivers.

May have been the perfect place
for him to grow.

As summer sun shines
and cool rainy winters,

allowed him to become
this great little fellow I know!

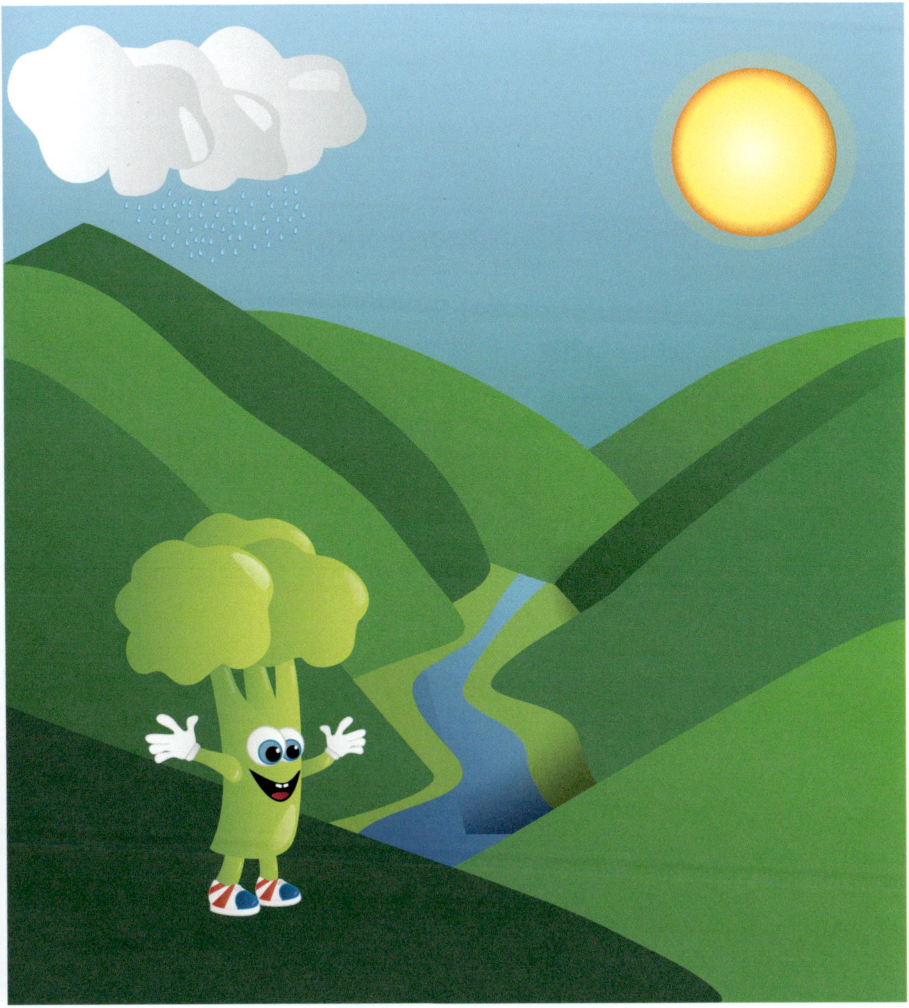

One day Pauly's mommy explained:

"We have been around
for about 2,000 years.

During The Roman Empire,
the Italian Broccoli premiered.

In a flash,
broccolis were served on family's dinners.

They tasted so delicious,
everyone cheered."

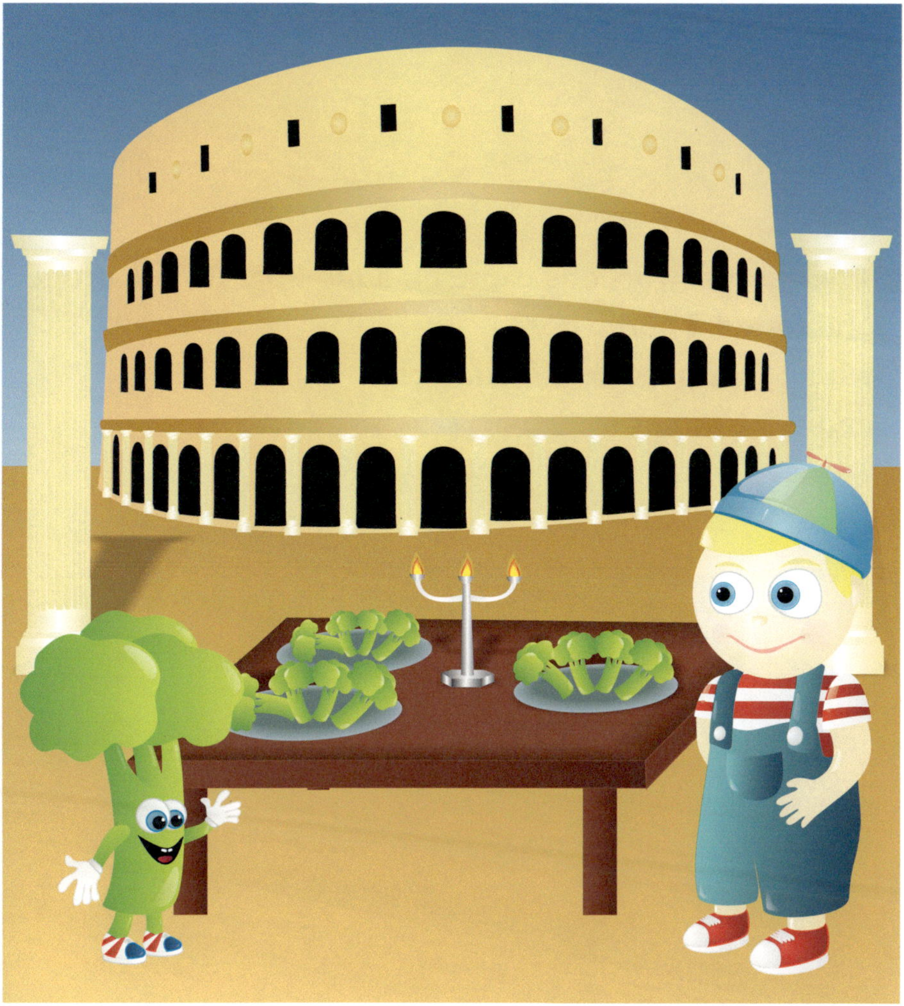

Then some broccolis came on a big boat from Europe
and found a home here,
where they grew lots of babies
and were happy to live near!

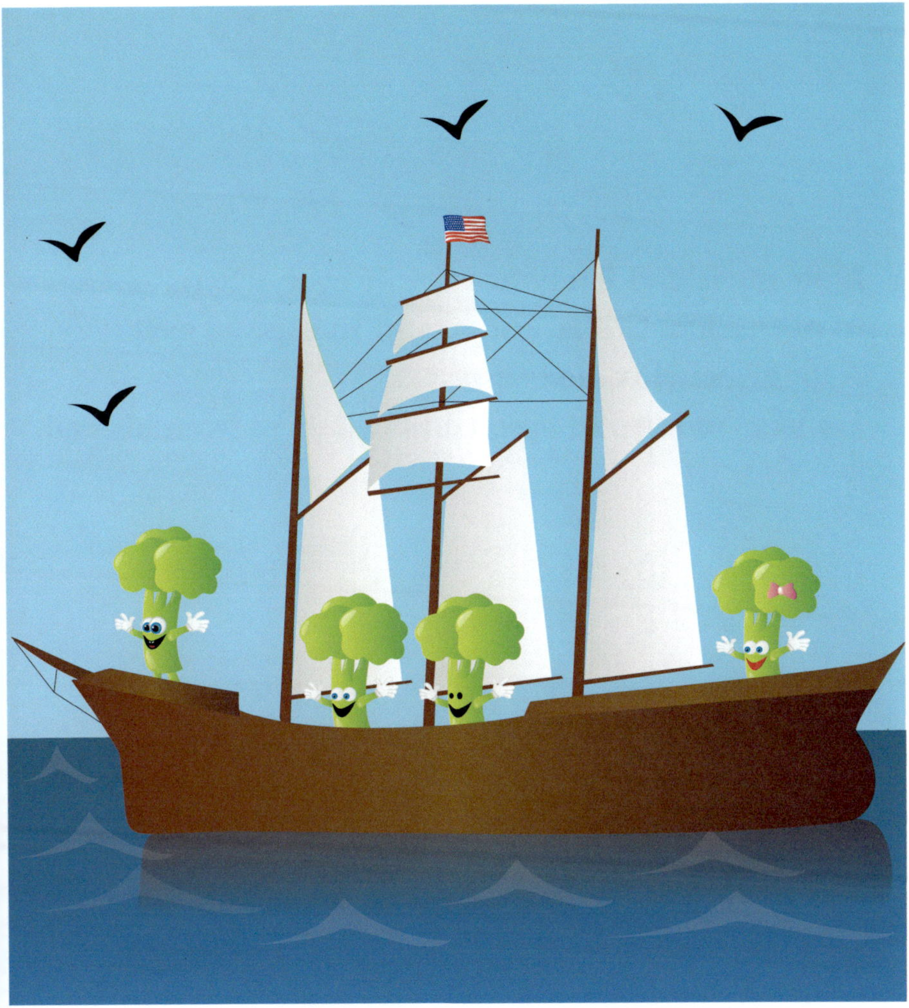

Now my friend Pauly has family everywhere,
in places like China, India, and Europe as well.
A lot of cousins, he is aware...
He likes to keep in touch and call them from his cell!

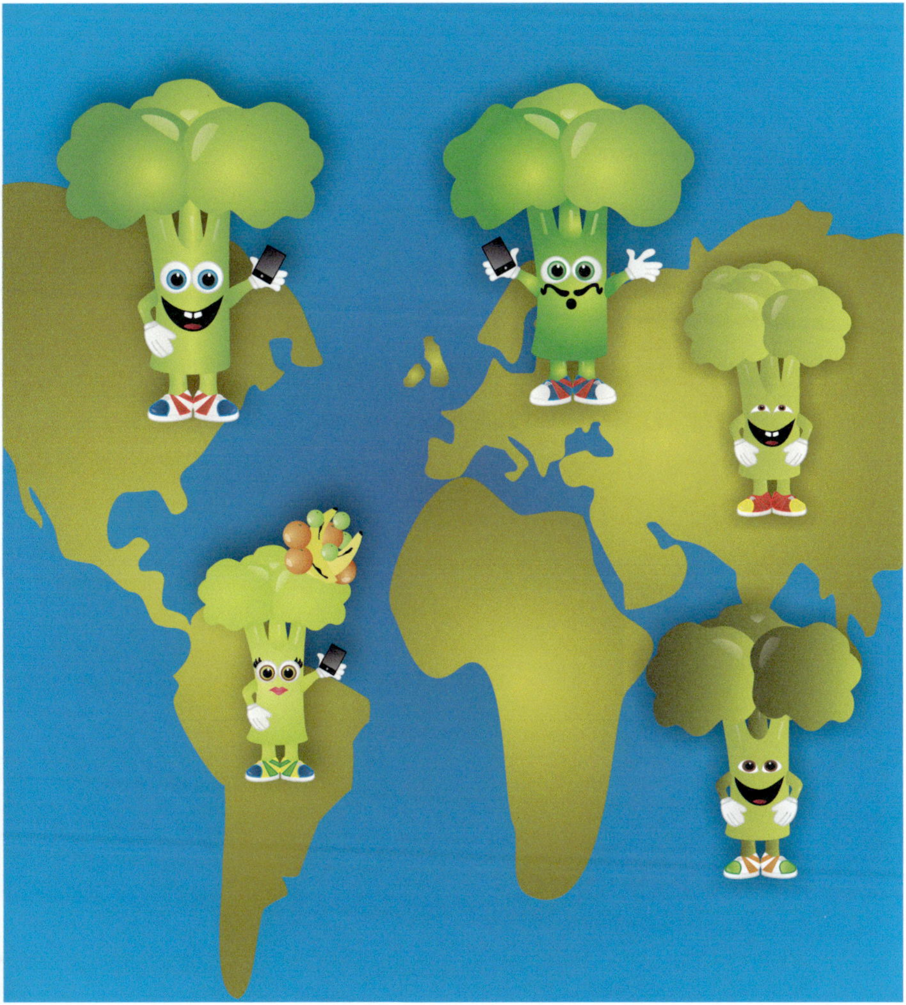

Some broccolis with big heads and thick stalks,
and some with many heads and little thin stalks.
Some green, some in yellow colors,
and even some with purple casts...
All delightful and a blast!!!

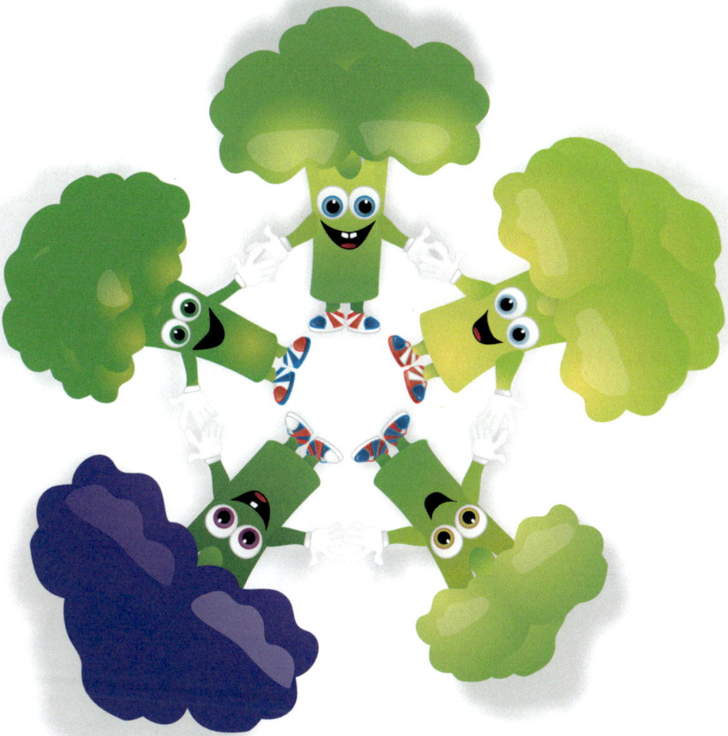

My little buddy Pauly is high in vitamin C,
which is very good for me.
And so, when I eat broccoli...
I get to go to the park and give the ball a kick,
as vitamins won't let me stay home sick!

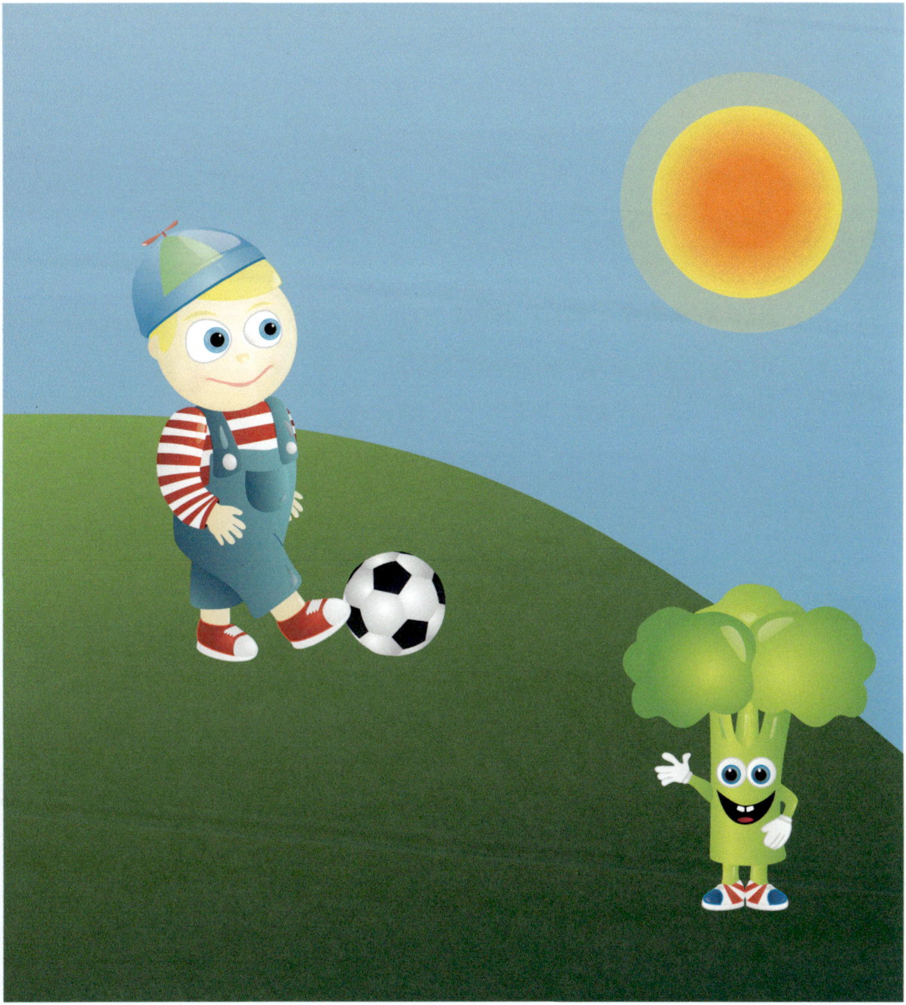

My friend Pauly told me
and very well explained,
how I can get a lot of energy
just by having a good taste, he sustained.

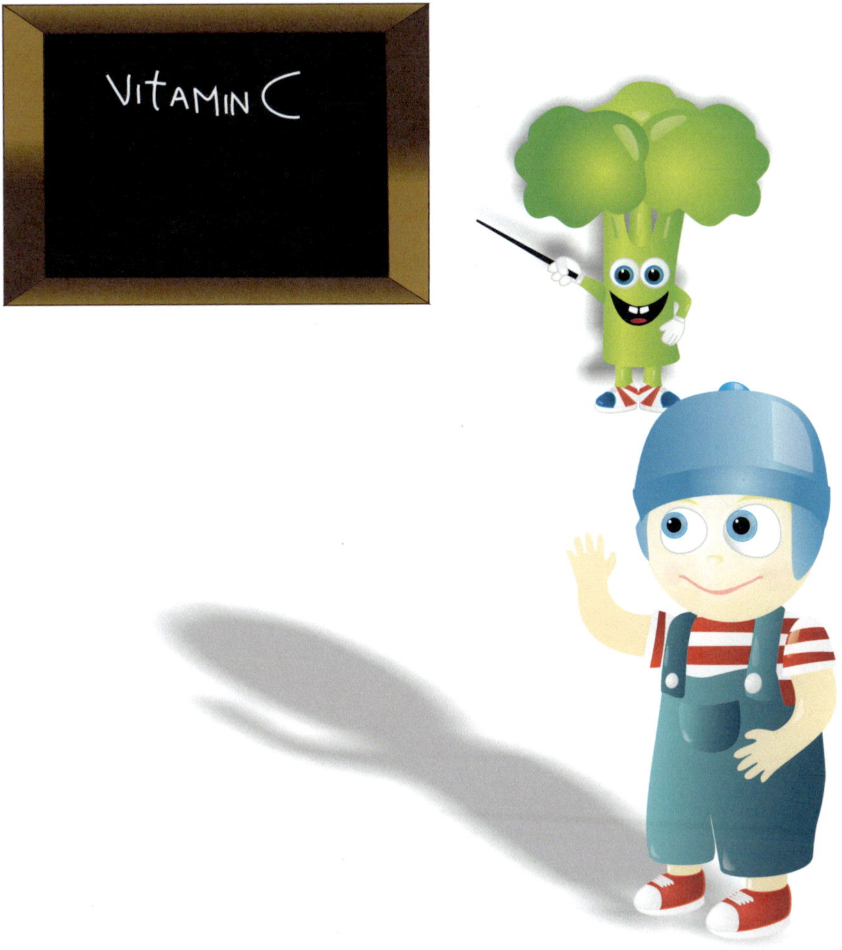
VITAMIN C

My mom can include broccoli in every meal,
in my breakfast, in my lunch, or in my dinner...
It is surreal!

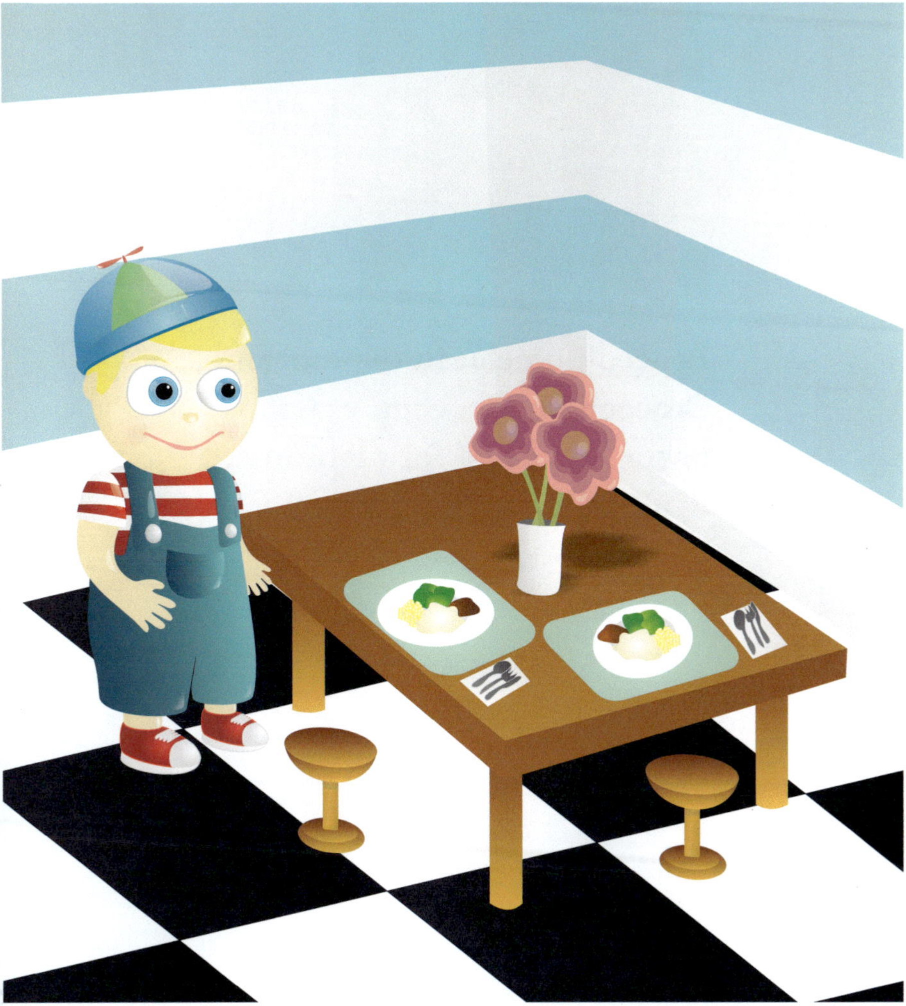

Broccoli omelet in the morning,
Broccoli cheese soup at noon,
pasta primavera for nighttime,
while enjoying the moon!!!

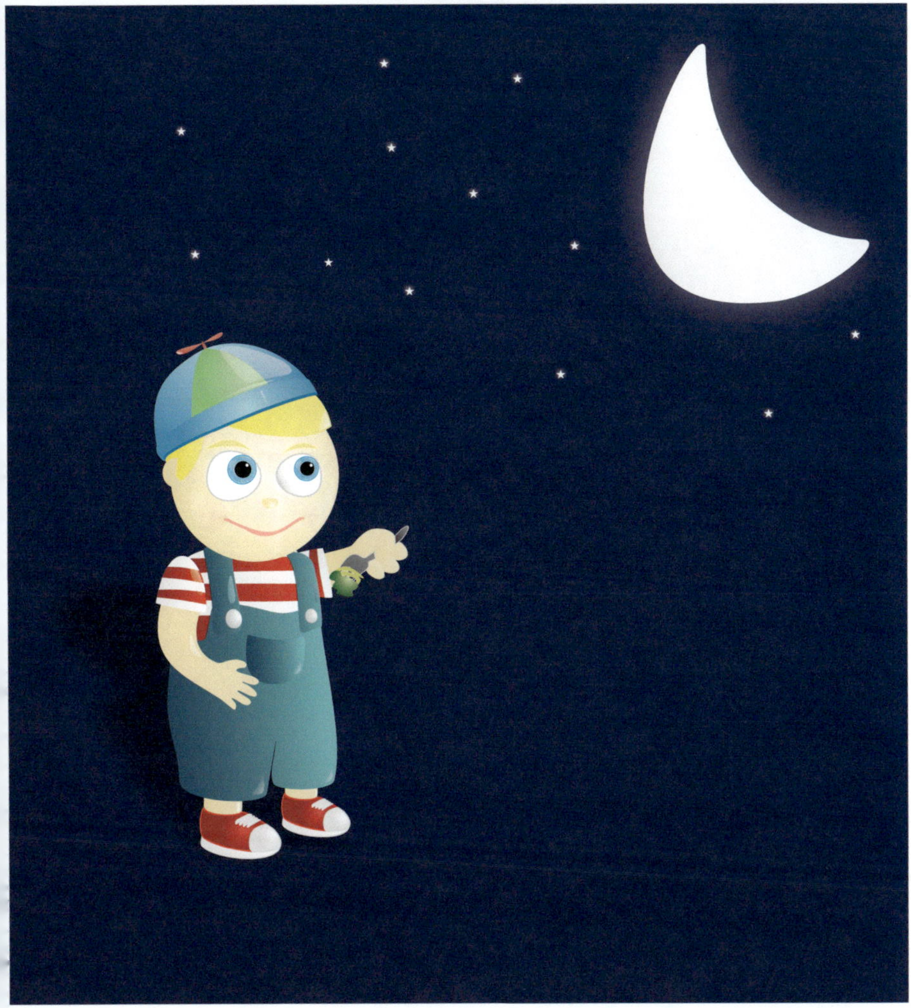

You can eat it raw,
like grandpa!
You might eat it steamed,
as the other night I dreamed!
You could even eat it boiled,
but hurry!!!
Don't let it get spoiled!

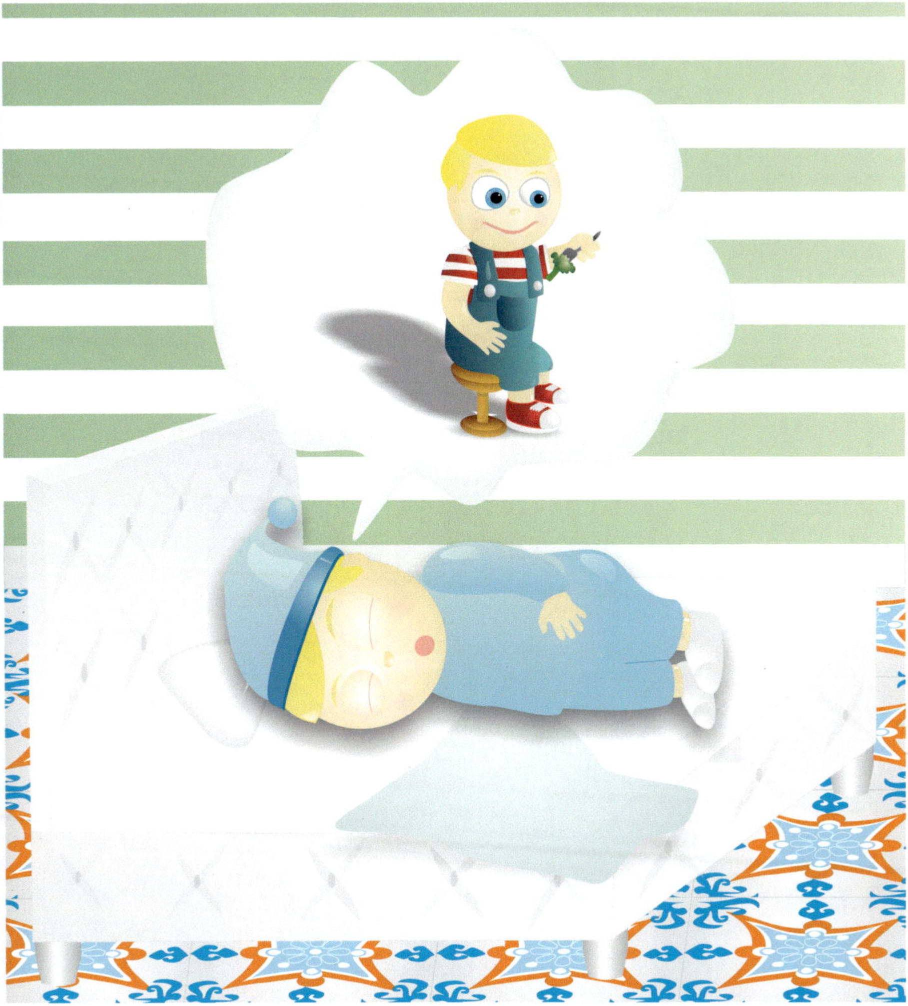

Whichever way it may be,
broccoli is so good for me!
Pauly is so much fun and sweet,
he makes my life complete!!!

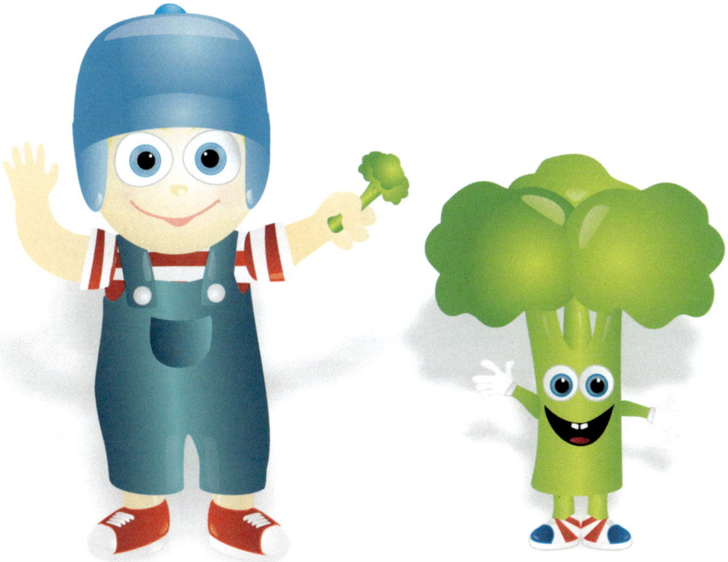

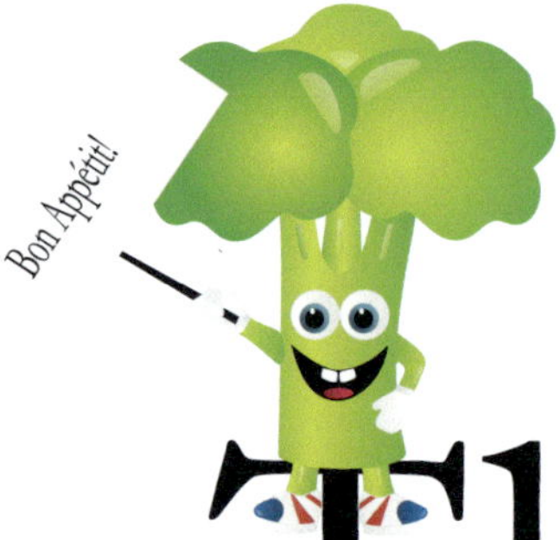

The End

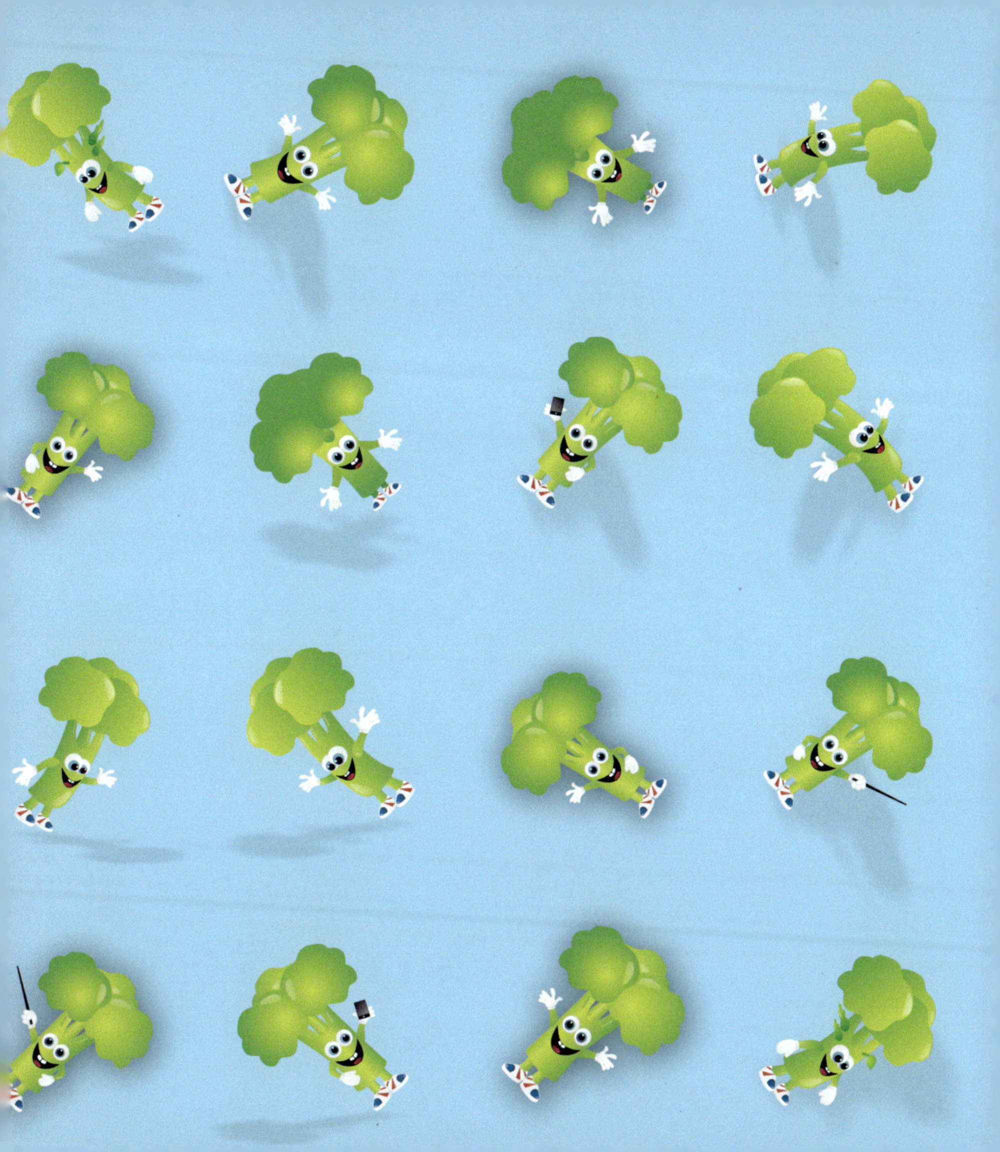

Made in the USA
Monee, IL
05 November 2026

67386144R00024